SculptHer:
A 12-Week Body Sculpting Plan for Women

Introduction:

Welcome to SculptHer, a comprehensive 12-week body sculpting plan designed specifically for women who want to transform their bodies, boost their confidence, and embrace a healthier lifestyle. Whether you're a beginner or an experienced fitness enthusiast, this ebook will guide you through a series of workouts, nutrition tips, and mindset strategies to help you achieve your fitness goals.

Week 1-4: Foundation Building

- Understanding Body Composition

Understanding body composition is crucial for effective body sculpting. Body composition refers to the proportion of fat, muscle, bone, and other tissues in your body. Here's why it's important and how it relates to body sculpting:

1. Fat vs. Muscle: Body composition analysis helps differentiate between fat mass and lean mass (muscle, bones, organs, etc.). While some fat is necessary for bodily functions, excessive fat can lead to health issues and affect your body shape. Muscle, on the other hand, contributes to a toned and defined physique.

2. Setting Realistic Goals: Knowing your body composition allows you to set realistic goals. Instead of solely focusing on weight loss, you can aim to decrease body fat percentage while maintaining or increasing lean muscle mass, leading to a more sculpted appearance.

3. Tracking Progress: Monitoring changes in body composition provides a more accurate reflection of your progress than just tracking weight. For example, even if the scale doesn't budge, a decrease in body fat percentage and an increase in muscle mass indicate positive changes in body composition.

4. Tailoring Workouts and Nutrition: Understanding your body composition helps tailor your workout and nutrition plan to your specific needs. For instance, if you have a higher body fat percentage, your focus might be on fat loss through a combination of strength training, cardio, and a calorie-controlled diet. If you're looking to build muscle, you'll need to prioritize resistance training and adequate protein intake.

5. Motivation and Accountability: Seeing improvements in body composition can be highly motivating and reinforce your commitment to your fitness journey. Regular body composition assessments provide accountability and help you stay on track towards your goals.

Methods for Assessing Body Composition:

- Body Measurements: Waist circumference, hip circumference, and skinfold measurements can provide estimates of body fat percentage.

- Bioelectrical Impedance Analysis (BIA): This method measures body composition by sending a low-level electrical current through the body.

- Dual-Energy X-ray Absorptiometry (DEXA): Considered one of the most accurate methods, DEXA scans measure bone density, fat mass, and lean mass.

- Air Displacement Plethysmography (Bod Pod): This method measures body composition by determining body volume and density.

By understanding your body composition and regularly assessing it throughout your body sculpting journey, you can make informed decisions and optimize your efforts towards achieving your desired physique.

- Setting Realistic Goals

Setting realistic goals is essential for any fitness program to ensure long-term success and motivation. Here's how to set realistic goals in a fitness program:

1. Be Specific: Clearly define what you want to achieve. Instead of a vague goal like "getting in shape," specify what "getting in shape" means to you, such as losing a certain amount of body fat, increasing muscle mass, or improving cardiovascular endurance.

2. Make Them Measurable: Goals should be quantifiable so that you can track your progress. For example, instead of saying "I want to lose weight," specify how much weight you want to lose within a certain timeframe.

3. Achievable: Set goals that are within your reach but still require effort. Consider your current fitness level, lifestyle, and resources. If you're new to exercise, aiming to run a marathon in a month may not be realistic, but completing a 5K race could be achievable.

4. Relevant: Ensure that your goals align with your overall fitness aspirations and personal values. Choose goals that are meaningful to you and will contribute to your overall well-being and happiness.

5. Time-Bound: Set a deadline for achieving your goals. Having a timeframe creates a sense of urgency and helps you stay focused and motivated. However, make sure the deadline is realistic and allows enough time to make sustainable progress.

6. Break Them Down: Break larger goals into smaller, manageable milestones. This makes them less overwhelming and allows you to celebrate achievements along the way, keeping you motivated.

7. Adjust as Needed: Be flexible and willing to adjust your goals based on your progress, changing circumstances, and feedback from your body. It's okay to modify your goals as you learn more about what works best for you.

Example:
Instead of setting a broad goal like "lose weight," a more realistic and specific goal could be: "Lose 1-2 pounds per week over the next three months by following a balanced diet and exercising for at least 30 minutes, five days a week. By the end of the three months, I aim to have lost 12-24 pounds and feel stronger and more energized."

Remember, setting realistic goals sets you up for success by providing direction, motivation, and a sense of accomplishment as you progress through your fitness journey.

- Basic Nutrition Guidelines

In a sculpting program, nutrition plays a critical role in fueling your workouts, supporting muscle growth, and promoting fat loss. Here are some basic nutrition guidelines to follow:

1. Balanced Macronutrients: Ensure your diet includes a balance of carbohydrates, protein, and healthy fats. Carbohydrates provide energy for workouts, protein supports muscle repair and growth, and fats are essential for hormone production and overall health.

2. Adequate Protein Intake: Aim to consume enough protein to support muscle growth and repair. Good sources of protein include lean meats, poultry, fish, eggs, dairy products, legumes, tofu, and tempeh.

3. Complex Carbohydrates: Choose complex carbohydrates like whole grains, fruits, vegetables, and legumes, which provide sustained energy and fiber to keep you feeling full and satisfied.

4. Healthy Fats: Include sources of healthy fats such as avocados, nuts, seeds, olive oil, and fatty fish like salmon. These fats provide essential fatty acids and help keep you feeling satiated.

5. Portion Control: Pay attention to portion sizes to avoid overeating and consuming excess calories. Use tools like measuring cups, food scales, or visual cues to help estimate serving sizes.

6. Hydration: Drink plenty of water throughout the day to stay hydrated, support digestion, and optimize performance during workouts. Aim for at least 8-10 cups of water daily, or more if you're physically active.

7. Pre- and Post-Workout Nutrition: Fuel your workouts with a balanced meal or snack containing carbohydrates and protein to provide energy and support muscle recovery. After workouts, consume a combination of protein and carbohydrates to replenish glycogen stores and promote muscle repair.

8. Meal Timing: Aim to eat regular meals and snacks spaced evenly throughout the day to maintain stable blood sugar levels and provide your body with a steady source of nutrients.

9. Limit Processed Foods and Added Sugars: Minimize your intake of processed foods, sugary snacks, and beverages, as they provide empty calories and can hinder progress towards your sculpting goals.

10. Listen to Your Body: Pay attention to hunger and fullness cues, and eat mindfully to avoid unnecessary snacking or overeating. Adjust your nutrition plan based on your individual needs and goals.

Remember, nutrition is a key component of any sculpting program, and finding a balance that works for you is essential for long-term success. Consulting with a registered dietitian or nutritionist can provide personalized guidance tailored to your specific needs and goals.

- Full-Body Strength Training Workouts

Incorporating full-body strength workouts into your sculpting program can help build lean muscle mass, increase metabolism, and promote overall body definition. Here's a sample full-body strength workout routine:

Warm-Up:
- 5-10 minutes of dynamic stretching (arm circles, leg swings, hip circles)
- 5-10 minutes of light cardio (jogging, jumping jacks, high knees)

Workout:
Perform each exercise for the prescribed number of sets and repetitions with a rest period of 60-90 seconds between sets.

1. Squats:
   - Sets: 3
   - Reps: 10-12

- Technique: Stand with feet shoulder-width apart, toes slightly turned out. Lower your body as if sitting back into a chair, keeping your chest up and knees behind toes. Push through your heels to return to the starting position.

2. Push-Ups (or Modified Push-Ups):
   - Sets: 3
   - Reps: 8-12
   - Technique: Start in a plank position with hands shoulder-width apart. Lower your body until your chest nearly touches the ground, then push back up to the starting position. Keep your core engaged and back flat throughout the movement.

3. Dumbbell Lunges:
   - Sets: 3 (each leg)
   - Reps: 10-12
   - Technique: Hold a dumbbell in each hand, step forward with one foot, and lower your body until both knees are bent at a 90-degree angle. Keep your front knee aligned with your ankle and your back knee hovering just above the ground. Push through your front heel to return to the starting position.

4. Bent-Over Rows:
   - Sets: 3
   - Reps: 10-12
   - Technique: Hold a dumbbell in each hand with palms facing your body. Hinge at the hips, keeping your back flat and chest up, and let the dumbbells hang in front of you. Pull the dumbbells towards your chest, squeezing your shoulder blades together, then lower them back down with control.

5. Plank:
   - Sets: 3
   - Duration: Hold for 30-60 seconds
   - Technique: Start in a plank position with hands directly under shoulders and feet hip-width apart. Keep your body in a straight line from head to heels, engaging your core and glutes. Hold the position while breathing deeply.

6. Russian Twists:
   - Sets: 3
   - Reps: 12-15 (each side)
   - Technique: Sit on the floor with knees bent and feet lifted off the ground, leaning back slightly. Hold a dumbbell or medicine ball with both hands. Twist your torso to the right, bringing the weight towards the ground next to your hip, then twist to the left. Keep your core engaged throughout the movement.

Cool Down:
- 5-10 minutes of static stretching (hamstring stretch, quad stretch, chest stretch)

- Deep breathing and relaxation techniques

Remember to adjust the weight and intensity of the exercises based on your fitness level, and always consult with a fitness professional before starting any new workout program. Incorporating progressive overload by gradually increasing the weight or difficulty of the exercises over time will help you continue to challenge your muscles and make progress towards your sculpting goals.

- Cardiovascular Exercises For Fat Loss

Incorporating cardio exercises into your sculpting program can help increase calorie burn, accelerate fat loss, and improve cardiovascular health. Here are some effective cardio exercises to include:

1. High Intensity Interval Training (HIIT):
   - HIIT involves alternating between short bursts of high-intensity exercise and brief periods of rest or lower-intensity activity.
   - Example: Perform 30 seconds of all-out sprinting followed by 60 seconds of walking or jogging. Repeat for 10-15 minutes.

2. Circuit Training:
   - Combine strength training exercises with cardio intervals to create a challenging full-body workout.
   - Example: Perform a circuit of bodyweight exercises like jumping jacks, burpees, mountain climbers, and high knees with minimal rest between exercises.

3. Running or Jogging:
   - Running or jogging is a straightforward yet effective way to burn calories and improve cardiovascular endurance.
   - Vary your pace with intervals of faster running followed by periods of jogging or walking to increase intensity.

4. Cycling:
   - Whether on a stationary bike or outdoors, cycling is a low-impact cardio exercise that engages the lower body muscles while providing an effective cardiovascular workout.
   - Increase resistance or incorporate intervals of sprinting to challenge yourself.

5. Rowing:
   - Rowing is a full-body exercise that engages multiple muscle groups while providing a cardiovascular challenge.
   - Aim for a steady pace or incorporate intervals of high-intensity rowing followed by periods of rest or lighter rowing.

6. Jump Rope:

- Jumping rope is a high-intensity, calorie-burning exercise that can be done almost anywhere with minimal equipment.
   - Start with short intervals and gradually increase the duration as your stamina improves.

7. Swimming:
   - Swimming is a low-impact cardio exercise that provides a full-body workout while being gentle on the joints.
   - Mix up your strokes and incorporate intervals of higher intensity swimming to increase calorie burn.

8. Stair Climbing:
   - Climbing stairs is an excellent way to target the lower body muscles while elevating your heart rate.
   - Find a staircase or use a stair climber machine and vary your speed or step height for added intensity.

9. Kickboxing or Martial Arts:
   - Kickboxing or martial arts classes combine cardio and strength training in a fun and dynamic way.
   - Punching, kicking, and other martial arts movements provide a high-intensity workout that burns calories and improves coordination.

10. Dance Workouts:
   - Dance-based workouts like Zumba, hip-hop dance, or aerobic dance classes are a fun way to get your heart pumping while burning calories and improving coordination.

Incorporate a variety of cardio exercises into your sculpting program to keep your workouts engaging and effective. Aim for at least 150 minutes of moderate-intensity cardio or 75 minutes of vigorous-intensity cardio per week, combined with strength training and a balanced diet, to maximize fat loss and sculpt your body.

- Flexibility and Mobility Routines

Including flexibility and mobility routines in your sculpting program is crucial for improving range of motion, preventing injuries, and enhancing overall performance. Here's a sample routine you can incorporate:

Warm-Up:
Begin your flexibility and mobility routine with 5-10 minutes of light cardio, such as jogging in place or jumping jacks, to increase blood flow to your muscles and prepare your body for stretching.

Dynamic Stretching:

Perform dynamic stretches to improve flexibility and mobility through a range of motion. Complete each movement for 8-10 repetitions per side.

1. Arm Circles: Stand with feet shoulder-width apart and extend your arms out to the sides. Make small circles with your arms, gradually increasing the size of the circles with each repetition.
2. Leg Swings: Hold onto a stable surface for balance and swing one leg forward and backward, then side to side. Repeat on the other leg.
3. Hip Circles: Stand with feet hip-width apart and hands on hips. Circle your hips clockwise, then counterclockwise, focusing on smooth, controlled movements.
4. Torso Twists: Stand tall with feet hip-width apart and arms extended out to the sides. Twist your torso to the right, bringing your left hand across your body to touch your right hand. Return to the starting position and repeat on the other side.
5. Lunge with Rotation: Step forward into a lunge position, then twist your torso towards the front leg. Return to the starting position and repeat on the other side.

Static Stretching:
Hold each static stretch for 20-30 seconds, focusing on breathing deeply and relaxing into the stretch. Stretch both sides of the body equally.

1. Hamstring Stretch: Sit on the floor with one leg extended straight in front of you and the other leg bent with the sole of the foot against the inner thigh of the extended leg. Lean forward from your hips, reaching towards your toes.
2. Quad Stretch: Stand tall and grab one ankle with your hand, bringing your heel towards your glutes. Keep your knees close together and gently push your hips forward to deepen the stretch.
3. Chest Stretch: Stand with feet hip-width apart and interlace your fingers behind your back. Straighten your arms and lift them slightly, opening up your chest.
4. Shoulder Stretch: Extend one arm across your body at shoulder height and use your other hand to gently press the arm towards your chest. Repeat on the other side.
5. Calf Stretch: Stand facing a wall with one foot forward and the other foot back, both feet flat on the ground. Lean forward, keeping your back leg straight, until you feel a stretch in the calf of the back leg. Repeat on the other side.

Foam Rolling:
Finish your flexibility and mobility routine with 5-10 minutes of foam rolling to release tension in your muscles and improve tissue quality. Focus on areas of tightness or discomfort, such as the calves, hamstrings, quadriceps, glutes, and back.

Incorporate this flexibility and mobility routine into your sculpting program 2-3 times per week, either as a standalone session or before or after your strength workouts. Consistency is key to seeing improvements in flexibility, mobility, and overall performance.

Week 5-8: Muscle Definition

- Fine-Tuning Your Diet For Muscle Definition

Fine-tuning your diet for muscle definition involves optimizing your nutrition to support muscle growth while minimizing body fat. Here are some key principles to follow:

1. Adequate Protein Intake: Protein is essential for building and repairing muscle tissue. Aim to consume lean sources of protein with each meal, such as chicken breast, turkey, fish, lean beef, tofu, tempeh, legumes, and low-fat dairy products. Aim for approximately 1.2-2.0 grams of protein per kilogram of body weight per day, depending on your activity level and goals.

2. Balanced Macronutrients: Along with protein, ensure you're getting adequate amounts of carbohydrates and healthy fats to support overall energy levels and hormone function. Choose complex carbohydrates like whole grains, fruits, vegetables, and legumes, as well as sources of healthy fats like avocados, nuts, seeds, olive oil, and fatty fish.

3. Caloric Surplus or Deficit: To build muscle, you need to consume slightly more calories than your body burns (caloric surplus), while to promote fat loss and reveal muscle definition, you need to consume slightly fewer calories than your body burns (caloric deficit). Determine your calorie needs based on your activity level, metabolism, and goals, and adjust your intake accordingly.

4. Timing of Nutrient Intake: Distribute your macronutrients evenly throughout the day to support muscle repair and recovery. Aim to consume protein-rich meals or snacks every 3-4 hours to optimize muscle protein synthesis. Additionally, consuming carbohydrates before and after workouts can provide energy for exercise and replenish glycogen stores.

5. Focus on Nutrient-Dense Foods: Choose nutrient-dense foods that provide a wide range of vitamins, minerals, and antioxidants to support overall health and performance. Incorporate plenty of fruits, vegetables, whole grains, lean proteins, and healthy fats into your diet while minimizing processed foods, added sugars, and refined carbohydrates.

6. Hydration: Stay hydrated by drinking plenty of water throughout the day. Adequate hydration is essential for optimal muscle function, recovery, and overall performance. Aim for at least 8-10 cups of water per day, or more if you're physically active or in a hot climate.

7. Monitor Progress and Adjust as Needed: Keep track of your progress by regularly monitoring your body composition, strength gains, and performance in the gym. Adjust your nutrition plan as needed based on your results, feedback from your body, and any changes in your goals or lifestyle.

Remember that achieving muscle definition is a gradual process that requires consistency, patience, and dedication to both your diet and exercise regimen. Consult with a registered dietitian or nutritionist for personalized guidance tailored to your specific needs and goals.

- Targeted Strength Training For Muscle Definition

Targeted strength training routines can help enhance muscle definition by focusing on specific muscle groups and incorporating exercises that promote muscle hypertrophy (growth) and definition. Here's a sample targeted strength training routine for muscle definition:

Day 1: Upper Body

1. Bench Press:
   - Sets: 3
   - Reps: 8-12
   - Technique: Lie on a flat bench with a barbell or dumbbells, lower the weight towards your chest, then press it back up, engaging your chest, shoulders, and triceps.

2. Bent-Over Rows:
   - Sets: 3
   - Reps: 8-12
   - Technique: Hinge at the hips with a slight bend in the knees, hold a barbell or dumbbells with an overhand grip, pull the weight towards your lower ribs, squeezing your shoulder blades together.

3. Overhead Shoulder Press:
   - Sets: 3
   - Reps: 8-12
   - Technique: Stand or sit with a barbell or dumbbells at shoulder height, press the weight overhead, fully extending your arms, then lower it back down under control.

4. Dumbbell Bicep Curls:
   - Sets: 3
   - Reps: 10-15
   - Technique: Hold dumbbells at your sides with palms facing forward, curl the weights towards your shoulders, keeping your elbows close to your body, then lower them back down.

5. Tricep Dips (or Tricep Pushdowns):
   - Sets: 3
   - Reps: 10-15
   - Technique: Use parallel bars or a bench, lower your body by bending your elbows, then press back up, engaging your triceps. Alternatively, use a cable machine for tricep pushdowns.

Day 2: Lower Body
1. Squats:
   - Sets: 3
   - Reps: 8-12

- Technique: Stand with feet shoulder-width apart, lower your body as if sitting back into a chair, then press through your heels to return to the starting position, engaging your quadriceps, hamstrings, and glutes.

2. Deadlifts:
   - Sets: 3
   - Reps: 8-12
   - Technique: Stand with feet hip-width apart, hold a barbell or dumbbells with an overhand grip, hinge at the hips and lower the weight towards the ground, then drive through your heels to stand up, engaging your hamstrings, glutes, and lower back.

3. Lunges:
   - Sets: 3 (each leg)
   - Reps: 8-12
   - Technique: Step forward with one foot, lower your body until both knees are bent at a 90-degree angle, then press through your front heel to return to the starting position, alternating legs.

4. Romanian Deadlifts:
   - Sets: 3
   - Reps: 8-12
   - Technique: Hold a barbell or dumbbells with an overhand grip, hinge at the hips with a slight bend in the knees, lower the weight towards the ground while keeping your back flat, then return to the starting position by squeezing your glutes and hamstrings.

5. Calf Raises:
   - Sets: 3
   - Reps: 12-15
   - Technique: Stand on a step or platform with heels hanging off the edge, lower your heels towards the ground, then press through the balls of your feet to raise your heels as high as possible, engaging your calf muscles.

Day 3: Rest or Active Recovery
Take a rest day or engage in light activity such as walking, yoga, or stretching to promote recovery and reduce muscle soreness.

Day 4: Total Body Circuit
Perform a circuit of compound exercises targeting multiple muscle groups to maximize calorie burn and muscle engagement. Complete each exercise back-to-back with minimal rest between exercises. Repeat the circuit 2-3 times.

1. Dumbbell Thrusters:
   - Sets: 3
   - Reps: 10-12

- Technique: Hold dumbbells at shoulder height, squat down, then explosively press the weights overhead as you stand up.

2. Renegade Rows:
   - Sets: 3
   - Reps: 8-10 (each arm)
   - Technique: Hold dumbbells in a plank position, row one weight towards your hip while stabilizing with the opposite arm, then alternate sides.

3. Mountain Climbers:
   - Sets: 3
   - Reps: 20-30 (total)
   - Technique: Start in a plank position, drive one knee towards your chest, then quickly switch legs, alternating in a running motion.

4. Russian Twists:
   - Sets: 3
   - Reps: 12-15 (each side)
   - Technique: Sit on the floor with knees bent and feet lifted off the ground, hold a weight or medicine ball with both hands, twist your torso to the right, then to the left.

5. Plank with Shoulder Taps:
   - Sets: 3
   - Reps: 10-12 (each side)
   - Technique: Start in a plank position, stabilize your core, and tap your right hand to your left shoulder, then your left hand to your right shoulder, alternating sides.

Day 5: Rest or Active Recovery
Take another rest day or engage in light activity to allow your muscles to recover and repair.

Repeat this 5-day split throughout the week, adjusting the weight and intensity of the exercises as needed to challenge your muscles and promote muscle definition. Remember to prioritize proper nutrition, hydration, and recovery to support your strength training efforts and maximize results.

- High-Intensity Interval Training (HIIT) For Maximum Calorie Burn

High-Intensity Interval Training (HIIT) is an effective way to maximize calorie burn in a short amount of time. HIIT involves alternating between periods of high-intensity exercise and short rest or active recovery periods. Here are two sample HIIT routines for maximum calorie burn:

Routine 1: Bodyweight HIIT Circuit

Perform each exercise for 30 seconds, followed by 15 seconds of rest. Complete the circuit, rest for 1-2 minutes, then repeat for a total of 3-4 rounds.

1. Jumping Jacks: Start with your feet together and arms at your sides. Jump while spreading your legs and raising your arms overhead. Return to the starting position and repeat.
2. Burpees: Start in a standing position, squat down and place your hands on the ground, jump your feet back into a plank position, perform a push-up, jump your feet back to your hands, and explode upwards into a jump.
3. Mountain Climbers: Start in a plank position, bring one knee towards your chest, then quickly switch legs in a running motion, keeping your core engaged.
4. High Knees: Stand in place and quickly alternate lifting your knees towards your chest as high as possible, pumping your arms for momentum.
5. Jump Squats: Start in a squat position, explosively jump upwards, reaching your arms overhead, then land softly back into the squat position.
6. Plank Jacks: Start in a plank position, jump your feet out wide, then back together, keeping your core engaged and hips stable.
7. Squat Jumps: Start in a squat position, explode upwards into a jump, reaching your arms overhead, then land softly back into the squat position.
8. Bicycle Crunches: Lie on your back with your hands behind your head, bring one knee towards your chest while twisting your torso to bring the opposite elbow towards the knee, alternating sides in a cycling motion.

Routine 2: Cardio and Strength HIIT

Perform each exercise for 40 seconds, followed by 20 seconds of rest. Complete the circuit, rest for 1-2 minutes, then repeat for a total of 3-4 rounds.

1. Jump Rope: Perform continuous jumping rope for 40 seconds, focusing on maintaining a steady rhythm and engaging your arms.
2. Dumbbell Thrusters: Hold a pair of dumbbells at shoulder height, squat down, then explosively press the weights overhead as you stand up.
3. Squat Jumps: Perform explosive squat jumps, reaching your arms overhead at the top of the jump.
4. Mountain Climbers: Perform mountain climbers in a plank position, bringing your knees towards your chest in a running motion.
5. Box Jumps (or Step-Ups): Use a plyometric box or bench to perform box jumps, or perform step-ups with a higher intensity, alternating legs.
6. Battle Ropes: Hold onto battle ropes with both hands and perform waves, slams, or alternating waves for 40 seconds, engaging your upper body and core.
7. Jumping Lunges: Perform alternating jumping lunges, switching legs in mid-air and landing softly in a lunge position.
8. Plank Hold with Shoulder Taps: Hold a plank position while alternating tapping your shoulders with each hand, keeping your core stable and hips level.

These HIIT routines are designed to elevate your heart rate, burn calories, and improve cardiovascular fitness while incorporating both bodyweight and strength exercises for a total-body workout. Adjust the intensity and duration of the exercises based on your fitness level and goals, and always listen to your body, modifying as needed to maintain proper form and prevent injury.

- Incorporating Plyometric Exercises For Explosive Power

Incorporating plyometric exercises into your sculpting program can help increase power, explosiveness, and overall athleticism, while also contributing to muscle definition. Plyometrics involve quick, explosive movements that utilize the stretch-shortening cycle of muscles to generate force. Here are some plyometric exercises to add to your sculpting program:

1. Jump Squats:
   - Technique: Start in a squat position, then explode upwards into a jump, reaching your arms overhead. Land softly and immediately transition into the next squat.
   - Benefits: Targets the lower body muscles including quadriceps, hamstrings, and glutes, while also engaging the core and improving cardiovascular fitness.

2. Box Jumps:
   - Technique: Stand in front of a sturdy box or platform, squat down, then explode upwards into a jump, landing softly on top of the box with both feet. Step back down and repeat.
   - Benefits: Increases lower body power, strength, and explosiveness, while also improving coordination and balance.

3. Plyometric Push-Ups:
   - Technique: Start in a plank position with hands shoulder-width apart, lower your body towards the ground in a push-up, then explosively push off the ground with enough force to lift your hands off the ground. Land softly and immediately transition into the next repetition.
   - Benefits: Targets the chest, shoulders, and triceps, while also engaging the core and improving upper body power and strength.

4. Jumping Lunges:
   - Technique: Start in a lunge position with one foot forward and the other foot back, lower your body into a lunge, then explosively jump upwards and switch legs in mid-air, landing softly in a lunge position with the opposite foot forward.
   - Benefits: Targets the lower body muscles including quadriceps, hamstrings, and glutes, while also improving balance, coordination, and agility.

5. Tuck Jumps:
   - Technique: Stand with feet hip-width apart, squat down, then explode upwards into a jump, bringing your knees towards your chest in a tuck position. Land softly and immediately transition into the next repetition.

- Benefits: Increases lower body power, explosiveness, and agility, while also engaging the core and improving cardiovascular fitness.

6. Depth Jumps:
   - Technique: Stand on a sturdy box or platform, step off the box and immediately upon landing, explode upwards into a vertical jump. Focus on minimizing ground contact time between landing and takeoff.
   - Benefits: Improves lower body power, explosiveness, and reactive strength, while also enhancing coordination and balance.

Incorporate plyometric exercises into your sculpting program 2-3 times per week, either as standalone workouts or as part of your strength training routine. Start with 2-3 sets of 8-12 repetitions for each exercise, focusing on explosive movement and proper form. Gradually increase the intensity, volume, and complexity of the exercises as your strength and proficiency improve. Always warm up thoroughly before performing plyometric exercises and listen to your body, modifying as needed to prevent injury.

- Recovery Techniques To Prevent Overtraining

Recovery is essential to prevent overtraining and support optimal performance and progress in your sculpting program. Here are some strategies to incorporate into your routine:

1. Rest Days: Schedule regular rest days into your week to allow your muscles time to repair and recover. Aim for at least one or two days of complete rest per week, where you engage in light activity or relaxation instead of intense exercise.

2. Sleep: Prioritize quality sleep to support muscle recovery, hormone regulation, and overall health. Aim for 7-9 hours of uninterrupted sleep each night, and establish a consistent sleep schedule to optimize recovery.

3. Nutrition: Fuel your body with nutrient-rich foods to support recovery and muscle repair. Consume a balance of carbohydrates, protein, and healthy fats, and prioritize post-workout nutrition to replenish glycogen stores and promote muscle protein synthesis.

4. Hydration: Stay hydrated throughout the day to support optimal performance and recovery. Drink water before, during, and after workouts, and pay attention to signs of dehydration such as thirst, dry mouth, and dark urine.

5. Foam Rolling and Stretching: Incorporate foam rolling and stretching into your routine to reduce muscle tension, improve flexibility, and enhance recovery. Spend time targeting areas of tightness or soreness, and perform gentle stretching exercises to promote blood flow and range of motion.

6. Active Recovery: Engage in low-intensity activities such as walking, cycling, swimming, or yoga on rest days to promote blood flow, reduce muscle stiffness, and enhance recovery without adding additional stress to your body.

7. Massage and Bodywork: Consider incorporating massage therapy, acupuncture, or other forms of bodywork into your routine to alleviate muscle tension, reduce inflammation, and promote relaxation.

8. Stress Management: Manage stress levels through relaxation techniques such as deep breathing, meditation, or mindfulness practices. Chronic stress can negatively impact recovery and performance, so prioritize activities that promote mental and emotional well-being.

9. Progressive Overload: Avoid overtraining by gradually increasing the intensity, duration, and frequency of your workouts over time. Listen to your body, and allow for adequate recovery between sessions to prevent fatigue and injury.

10. Listen to Your Body: Pay attention to signs of overtraining such as persistent fatigue, decreased performance, irritability, and increased susceptibility to illness. If you experience these symptoms, consider scaling back your training volume or intensity, and prioritize rest and recovery until you feel rejuvenated.

By incorporating these recovery strategies into your sculpting program, you can optimize your performance, reduce the risk of overtraining, and support long-term progress towards your fitness goals. Remember that recovery is just as important as training itself, so prioritize self-care and listen to your body's signals.

Week 9-12: Sculpting and Shaping

- Advanced Nutrition Strategies For Sculpting

Advanced nutrition strategies can help optimize your sculpting efforts by fine-tuning your diet to support muscle growth, fat loss, and overall performance.

Here are some advanced nutrition tips for sculpting:

1. Periodized Nutrition: Align your nutrition plan with your training cycles by adjusting your calorie and macronutrient intake based on your goals and training intensity. For example, consume more carbohydrates and calories on heavy training days to fuel workouts and support muscle growth, and reduce intake on rest days to promote fat loss and recovery.

2. Nutrient Timing: Strategically time your meals and snacks around your workouts to maximize performance and recovery. Consume a balanced meal containing protein and carbohydrates within 1-2 hours before and after workouts to provide energy, support muscle repair, and replenish glycogen stores.

3. Macronutrient Cycling: Cycle your intake of carbohydrates and fats based on your training schedule and goals. Increase carbohydrate intake on training days to fuel workouts and support muscle glycogen replenishment, and reduce carbohydrate intake on rest days to promote fat burning and metabolic flexibility.

4. Protein Pacing: Distribute your protein intake evenly throughout the day to optimize muscle protein synthesis and support muscle repair and growth. Aim for a consistent intake of high-quality protein sources with each meal and snack, and consider consuming a protein-rich snack before bedtime to support overnight muscle recovery.

5. Targeted Supplementation: Consider incorporating targeted supplements into your regimen to enhance performance, recovery, and nutrient intake. Examples include whey protein powder, branched-chain amino acids (BCAAs), creatine, beta-alanine, caffeine, and fish oil. Consult with a healthcare professional or registered dietitian before adding supplements to your routine to ensure they are safe and appropriate for your individual needs.

6. Hydration Strategies: Stay hydrated by consuming adequate fluids throughout the day, paying attention to both water intake and electrolyte balance. Adjust your fluid intake based on sweat rate, environmental conditions, and training duration and intensity. Consider incorporating electrolyte-rich beverages or sports drinks during intense or prolonged workouts to maintain hydration and performance.

7. Tracking and Monitoring: Keep track of your dietary intake, training progress, and body composition changes to identify patterns, make adjustments, and optimize your nutrition plan over time. Use food journals, mobile apps, or tracking tools to monitor calorie and macronutrient intake, and consider regular assessments such as body measurements, body fat percentage, and performance tests to track progress and adjust your plan accordingly.

8. Individualization: Tailor your nutrition plan to your specific needs, preferences, and goals. Experiment with different dietary approaches, meal timing strategies, and nutrient ratios to find what works best for you in terms of performance, satiety, and adherence. Listen to your body's hunger and fullness cues, and prioritize foods that nourish and energize you while supporting your sculpting goals.

By implementing these advanced nutrition strategies, you can optimize your diet to support muscle definition, fat loss, and overall performance, while promoting long-term health and well-being. Experiment with different approaches, listen to your body, and seek guidance from qualified professionals to create a personalized nutrition plan that works best for you.

- Sculpting Specific Muscle Groups For A Toned Physique

To sculpt specific areas of your body for a toned appearance, it's important to combine targeted strength training exercises with a balanced diet and overall fitness routine. Here are some tips for targeting common trouble areas:

1. Abs/Core:
   - Incorporate exercises like planks, crunches, Russian twists, bicycle crunches, and leg raises to strengthen and define your abdominal muscles.
   - Focus on full-body exercises like squats, deadlifts, and overhead presses, which also engage the core muscles for stability and strength.

2. Arms:
   - Include exercises like bicep curls, tricep dips, overhead tricep extensions, hammer curls, and tricep pushdowns to target the biceps and triceps.
   - Incorporate compound exercises such as push-ups, bench presses, and rows, which engage multiple muscle groups including the arms.

3. Legs/Buttocks:
   - Perform exercises like squats, lunges, deadlifts, leg presses, and step-ups to strengthen and sculpt the quadriceps, hamstrings, and glutes.
   - Incorporate plyometric exercises like jump squats, box jumps, and lunges with a hop to increase power and definition in the lower body.

4. Back:
   - Include exercises like pull-ups, lat pulldowns, bent-over rows, seated rows, and reverse flyes to target the muscles of the upper and middle back.
   - Focus on exercises that improve posture and stability, such as face pulls and band pull-aparts, to enhance back definition and function.

5. Chest:
   - Perform exercises like push-ups, chest presses, dumbbell flyes, cable crossovers, and chest dips to target the muscles of the chest.
   - Incorporate incline and decline variations of pressing exercises to target different areas of the chest for balanced development.

6. Shoulders:
   - Include exercises like overhead presses, lateral raises, front raises, rear delt flyes, and upright rows to target the muscles of the shoulders.
   - Focus on maintaining proper form and range of motion to effectively target the deltoid muscles and create definition in the shoulders.

In addition to targeted strength training exercises, it's important to maintain a balanced diet that supports your fitness goals. Focus on consuming lean protein, complex carbohydrates, healthy fats, and plenty of fruits and vegetables to fuel your workouts and promote muscle growth and recovery.

Consistency is key when it comes to sculpting specific areas of the body. Aim to incorporate targeted strength training exercises into your routine at least 2-3 times per week, and gradually increase the intensity and difficulty of your workouts over time. Remember to listen to your body, rest when needed, and stay hydrated to support optimal performance and recovery.

- Circuit Training For Endurance and Muscle Definition

Circuit training routines are an excellent way to improve endurance, build muscle definition, and burn calories effectively. Here's a sample circuit training routine that combines strength and cardiovascular exercises to target multiple muscle groups while increasing endurance:

Warm-Up:
Begin with 5-10 minutes of dynamic stretching and light cardio, such as jogging in place, jumping jacks, or arm circles, to prepare your body for the workout.

Circuit:
Perform each exercise for 45-60 seconds, followed by 15-30 seconds of rest. Complete the entire circuit without resting between exercises. Rest for 1-2 minutes at the end of the circuit, then repeat for a total of 3-4 rounds.

1. Bodyweight Squats:
   - Technique: Stand with feet shoulder-width apart, lower your body into a squat position by bending your knees and pushing your hips back, then return to the starting position.
   - Benefits: Targets the quadriceps, hamstrings, glutes, and core muscles while improving lower body strength and endurance.

2. Push-Ups:
   - Technique: Start in a plank position with hands shoulder-width apart, lower your body towards the ground by bending your elbows, then push back up to the starting position.
   - Benefits: Targets the chest, shoulders, triceps, and core muscles while improving upper body strength and endurance.

3. Walking Lunges:
   - Technique: Step forward with one leg and lower your body until both knees are bent at a 90-degree angle, then push off the front foot to return to the starting position and repeat with the other leg.
   - Benefits: Targets the quadriceps, hamstrings, glutes, and calf muscles while improving lower body strength, balance, and coordination.

4. Plank with Shoulder Taps:
   - Technique: Start in a plank position with hands directly under shoulders, stabilize your core and tap your right hand to your left shoulder, then your left hand to your right shoulder, alternating sides.

  - Benefits: Engages the core, shoulder stabilizers, and oblique muscles while improving core strength and stability.

5. Jumping Jacks:
  - Technique: Start with feet together and arms at your sides, jump while spreading your legs and raising your arms overhead, then return to the starting position and repeat.
  - Benefits: Raises heart rate, improves cardiovascular endurance, and engages the entire body in a dynamic movement.

6. Russian Twists:
  - Technique: Sit on the floor with knees bent and feet lifted off the ground, hold a weight or medicine ball with both hands, twist your torso to the right, then to the left, while keeping your core engaged.
  - Benefits: Targets the oblique muscles, improves rotational strength and stability, and enhances core definition.

Cool Down:
Finish with 5-10 minutes of static stretching, focusing on the major muscle groups worked during the circuit, to promote flexibility and reduce muscle soreness.

Incorporate this circuit training routine into your workout regimen 2-3 times per week to improve endurance, increase muscle definition, and boost overall fitness. Adjust the intensity, duration, and difficulty of the exercises based on your fitness level and goals, and remember to listen to your body and rest as needed.

- Incorporating Resistance Bands and Bodyweight Exercises

Incorporating resistance bands and bodyweight exercises into your sculpting phase can effectively target and tone muscles while also improving strength, endurance, and flexibility. Here's how you can integrate bands and bodyweight exercises into your sculpting routine:

Warm-Up:
Start with a dynamic warm-up to prepare your muscles and joints for exercise. Perform movements such as arm circles, leg swings, hip circles, and bodyweight squats to increase blood flow and mobility.

Main Workout:

1. Resistance Band Squats:
  - Technique: Stand on the resistance band with feet shoulder-width apart, hold the handles at shoulder height, squat down by bending your knees and pushing your hips back, then return to the starting position.
  - Benefits: Targets the quadriceps, hamstrings, glutes, and core muscles while providing resistance throughout the movement.

2. Push-Ups with Resistance Band:
   - Technique: Loop the resistance band around your back and hold the ends in each hand, perform push-ups with the band providing resistance against your chest and arms.
   - Benefits: Engages the chest, shoulders, triceps, and core muscles while adding resistance to increase muscle activation and definition.

3. Resistance Band Rows:
   - Technique: Anchor the resistance band to a sturdy object at chest height, hold the handles with palms facing each other, retract your shoulder blades and pull the band towards your chest, then return to the starting position.
   - Benefits: Targets the muscles of the upper back, including the latissimus dorsi, rhomboids, and rear deltoids, to improve posture and upper body definition.

4. Glute Bridges with Resistance Band:
   - Technique: Lie on your back with knees bent and feet hip-width apart, place the resistance band above your knees, lift your hips towards the ceiling by squeezing your glutes, then lower back down.
   - Benefits: Activates the glutes, hamstrings, and lower back muscles to improve hip stability and enhance lower body definition.

5. Resistance Band Bicep Curls:
   - Technique: Stand on the resistance band with feet hip-width apart, hold the handles with palms facing upwards, curl the band towards your shoulders by contracting your biceps, then lower back down.
   - Benefits: Targets the biceps muscles to increase arm definition and strength while providing constant tension throughout the movement.

6. Plank with Resistance Band Leg Lifts:
   - Technique: Start in a plank position with the resistance band around your ankles, stabilize your core and lift one leg off the ground, then return to the starting position and repeat with the other leg.
   - Benefits: Engages the core, glutes, and hip stabilizers to improve balance, stability, and lower body definition.

Cool Down:
Finish with a cooldown consisting of static stretching exercises to promote flexibility and reduce muscle tension. Focus on stretching the major muscle groups worked during the workout, holding each stretch for 15-30 seconds.

Incorporate this resistance band and bodyweight workout into your sculpting phase 2-3 times per week, allowing at least one day of rest between sessions to allow for recovery. Adjust the resistance level of the bands and the intensity of the exercises based on your fitness level and goals, and listen to your body to avoid overtraining.

Bonus Content:

- Sample Meal Plans and Recipes

Here's a sample meal plan for body sculpting, along with some simple and nutritious recipes:

Meal Plan:

Day 1:
- Breakfast: Scrambled eggs with spinach and tomatoes, whole grain toast
- Snack: Greek yogurt with berries and almonds
- Lunch: Grilled chicken breast with quinoa salad (quinoa, cucumber, cherry tomatoes, feta cheese, lemon vinaigrette)
- Snack: Carrot sticks with hummus
- Dinner: Baked salmon with roasted sweet potatoes and steamed broccoli

Day 2:
- Breakfast: Overnight oats with almond milk, chia seeds, sliced banana, and a drizzle of honey
- Snack: Apple slices with peanut butter
- Lunch: Turkey and avocado wrap with whole grain tortilla, mixed greens, and mustard
- Snack: Cottage cheese with pineapple chunks
- Dinner: Lean beef stir-fry with mixed vegetables (bell peppers, onions, snap peas) served over brown rice

Day 3:
- Breakfast: Greek yogurt parfait with granola and mixed berries
- Snack: Handful of mixed nuts
- Lunch: Quinoa salad with chickpeas, roasted vegetables (zucchini, bell peppers, eggplant), and balsamic vinaigrette
- Snack: Celery sticks with almond butter
- Dinner: Grilled shrimp skewers with grilled asparagus and a side salad (mixed greens, cherry tomatoes, cucumber) with vinaigrette dressing

Recipes:

1. Quinoa Salad:
   - Cook quinoa according to package instructions and let it cool.
   - In a bowl, mix cooked quinoa with diced cucumber, halved cherry tomatoes, crumbled feta cheese, chopped fresh parsley, and a squeeze of lemon juice. Season with salt and pepper to taste.
   - Drizzle with olive oil and toss to combine. Serve chilled.

2. Turkey and Avocado Wrap:
   - Spread mustard over a whole grain tortilla.
   - Layer sliced turkey breast, sliced avocado, mixed greens, and any other desired toppings
(e.g., tomato, cucumber, onion).
   - Roll up the tortilla tightly and cut in half. Serve with carrot sticks or a side salad.

3. Baked Salmon:
   - Preheat oven to 375°F (190°C). Place salmon fillets on a baking sheet lined with parchment
paper.
   - Drizzle salmon with olive oil and season with salt, pepper, and any desired herbs or spices
(such as dill or lemon zest).
   - Bake for 12-15 minutes, or until salmon is cooked through and flakes easily with a fork.
Serve with roasted sweet potatoes and steamed broccoli.

4. Overnight Oats:
   - In a jar or bowl, combine rolled oats, almond milk, chia seeds, sliced banana, and a drizzle of
honey. Stir well to combine.
   - Cover and refrigerate overnight, or for at least 4 hours, to allow the oats to soften and absorb
the liquid.
   - Before serving, top with additional sliced banana, berries, and a sprinkle of granola for added
crunch.

These meal ideas and recipes provide a balance of protein, carbohydrates, and healthy fats to
support muscle growth, fat loss, and overall health during your body sculpting journey. Feel free
to customize the portion sizes and ingredients to fit your individual dietary preferences and
calorie needs.

- Grocery Shopping List

Here's a sample grocery shopping list for body sculpting:

Protein Sources:
1. Chicken breast
2. Turkey breast
3. Salmon fillets
4. Lean beef (such as sirloin or flank steak)
5. Eggs
6. Greek yogurt
7. Cottage cheese
8. Tofu or tempeh

Carbohydrate Sources:

1. Quinoa
2. Brown rice
3. Sweet potatoes
4. Oats (rolled or steel-cut)
5. Whole grain bread or wraps
6. Fresh fruits (such as berries, apples, bananas)
7. Vegetables (such as spinach, broccoli, kale, bell peppers, carrots)

Healthy Fats:
1. Avocado
2. Nuts (almonds, walnuts, cashews)
3. Seeds (chia seeds, flaxseeds, pumpkin seeds)
4. Olive oil or avocado oil
5. Nut butter (peanut butter, almond butter)

Dairy and Alternatives:
1. Milk (dairy or plant-based)
2. Cheese (such as feta or low-fat mozzarella)
3. Unsweetened almond or coconut milk (for smoothies or cereal)
4. Soy or almond yogurt

Miscellaneous:
1. Beans and legumes (black beans, chickpeas, lentils)
2. Hummus
3. Herbs and spices (such as garlic, onion, cumin, paprika)
4. Fresh herbs (such as basil, cilantro, parsley)
5. Healthy condiments (mustard, salsa, balsamic vinegar)
6. Protein powder (whey, plant-based)

Snacks and Extras:
1. Berries (strawberries, blueberries, raspberries)
2. Hummus and veggie sticks (carrots, celery, cucumber)
3. Rice cakes
4. Dark chocolate (70% or higher cocoa content)
5. Protein bars (look for ones with minimal added sugars and ingredients)
6. Herbal tea or flavored sparkling water

This shopping list includes a variety of nutrient-dense foods to support muscle building, energy levels, and overall health during your body sculpting journey. Adjust quantities based on your individual needs and preferences, and aim to prioritize whole, minimally processed foods as much as possible.

- Progress Tracking Tools and Aids

Tracking your progress is essential for staying motivated and making adjustments to your sculpting program as needed. Here are some aids and methods you can use to track your progress effectively:

1. Body Measurements: Take measurements of key areas such as chest, waist, hips, arms, and thighs using a tape measure. Record these measurements regularly (e.g., every 2 weeks) to track changes in body composition and muscle definition.

2. Body Weight: Weigh yourself regularly using a reliable scale. Keep in mind that fluctuations in body weight can be influenced by factors such as hydration, glycogen stores, and muscle gain, so focus on long-term trends rather than daily fluctuations.

3. Progress Photos: Take photos of yourself from multiple angles (front, side, and back) in consistent lighting and clothing every few weeks. Compare these photos over time to visually track changes in muscle definition, fat loss, and overall physique.

4. Strength and Performance: Keep a workout journal or log to track your strength progress and performance in the gym. Record details such as exercises, sets, reps, weights lifted, and rest periods. Aim to progressively increase the intensity or volume of your workouts over time to stimulate muscle growth and adaptation.

5. Fitness Apps: Use fitness tracking apps or websites to log workouts, track nutrition, and monitor progress over time. Many apps offer features such as workout plans, progress charts, and community support to help you stay accountable and motivated.

6. Body Fat Percentage: Consider using methods such as skinfold calipers, bioelectrical impedance analysis (BIA) scales, or DEXA scans to estimate body fat percentage. While these methods may not be perfectly accurate, they can provide valuable information about changes in body composition over time.

7. Nutrition Tracking: Keep a food diary or use a nutrition tracking app to monitor your daily food intake and macronutrient distribution. Pay attention to factors such as calorie intake, protein intake, and overall food quality to support your sculpting goals.

8. Consistency and Compliance: Track your adherence to your sculpting program and consistency with nutrition and workouts. Set specific goals and benchmarks for yourself, and regularly evaluate your progress towards achieving them.

By using a combination of these progress tracking aids, you can effectively monitor your progress, stay motivated, and make informed decisions to optimize your sculpting program for the best results. Remember that progress takes time and consistency, so be patient and celebrate your achievements along the way.

- Troubleshooting Common Fitness Obstacles

Here are some common fitness obstacles and strategies to troubleshoot them:

1. Lack of Motivation: Identify your reasons for wanting to improve your fitness and set specific, achievable goals. Find activities you enjoy and vary your workouts to keep things interesting. Surround yourself with supportive friends or join a fitness community for accountability and encouragement.

2. Time Constraints: Prioritize exercise by scheduling it into your day like any other appointment. Consider shorter, high-intensity workouts or break up your exercise sessions into smaller chunks throughout the day. Look for opportunities to incorporate physical activity into your daily routine, such as taking the stairs or walking during phone calls.

3. Plateaus: Mix up your workouts by trying new exercises, changing the intensity or duration of your workouts, or incorporating different types of training (e.g., strength training, cardio, flexibility). Pay attention to your nutrition and sleep habits, as these can also impact your progress. Consider consulting with a fitness professional for personalized guidance and advice.

4. Injuries or Pain: Listen to your body and avoid pushing through pain or discomfort. If you experience an injury, seek appropriate medical attention and follow recommended treatment and rehabilitation protocols. Modify your workouts to accommodate any limitations or restrictions, focusing on exercises that don't aggravate your injury.

5. Nutrition Challenges: Plan and prepare your meals ahead of time to avoid relying on unhealthy options when you're busy or stressed. Focus on whole, nutrient-dense foods and aim for a balanced diet that includes lean protein, complex carbohydrates, healthy fats, and plenty of fruits and vegetables. Practice mindful eating and pay attention to hunger and fullness cues.

6. Stress and Mental Health: Incorporate stress-reducing activities into your routine, such as meditation, yoga, or deep breathing exercises. Prioritize self-care and make time for activities that help you relax and unwind. If you're struggling with mental health issues, seek support from a therapist, counselor, or support group.

7. Lack of Results: Be patient and realistic with your expectations, as progress takes time and consistency. Focus on non-scale victories such as improvements in strength, endurance, and overall well-being. Consider tracking your progress using measurements, photos, or

performance metrics to see changes over time. Evaluate your habits and make adjustments as needed to support your goals.

By addressing these common obstacles with proactive strategies and solutions, you can overcome challenges and stay on track with your fitness journey. Remember that consistency, patience, and persistence are key to long-term success.

- Tips For Maintaining Your Results Long-Term

Maintaining long-term body sculpting results requires a sustainable approach that emphasizes consistency, balance, and healthy habits. Here are some tips to help you maintain your progress over the long term:

1. Lifestyle Changes: Focus on making lasting lifestyle changes rather than quick fixes or temporary solutions. Adopt a balanced approach to nutrition, exercise, and self-care that you can maintain for the long term.

2. Consistent Exercise Routine: Stick to a regular exercise routine that includes a combination of strength training, cardiovascular exercise, and flexibility/mobility work. Aim for at least 150 minutes of moderate-intensity aerobic activity or 75 minutes of vigorous-intensity activity per week, along with 2-3 days of strength training.

3. Progressive Overload: Continue to challenge your muscles by gradually increasing the intensity, duration, or frequency of your workouts over time. Progressively overload your muscles with heavier weights, more repetitions, or more challenging exercises to stimulate ongoing improvements in strength and muscle definition.

4. Balanced Nutrition: Maintain a balanced and nutrient-rich diet that supports your fitness goals while also promoting overall health and well-being. Focus on whole, minimally processed foods such as lean proteins, whole grains, fruits, vegetables, healthy fats, and plenty of water. Practice portion control and moderation, and be mindful of your calorie intake to avoid overeating.

5. Mindful Eating: Pay attention to your hunger and fullness cues, and practice mindful eating to prevent mindless snacking or overindulging. Eat slowly, savor each bite, and tune in to your body's signals of hunger and satisfaction.

6. Regular Monitoring: Stay accountable by regularly monitoring your progress and adjusting your habits as needed. Track your workouts, nutrition, and body measurements to ensure you're staying on track with your goals. Celebrate your achievements and use setbacks as learning opportunities to make improvements.

7. Rest and Recovery: Prioritize adequate rest and recovery to allow your body to repair and rebuild muscle tissue. Aim for 7-9 hours of quality sleep per night, and incorporate rest days into your workout schedule to prevent burnout and reduce the risk of injury.

8. Healthy Coping Mechanisms: Find healthy ways to manage stress and cope with emotions without relying on food or unhealthy behaviors. Practice relaxation techniques such as deep breathing, meditation, yoga, or spending time outdoors to reduce stress and promote mental well-being.

9. Social Support: Surround yourself with supportive friends, family members, or workout buddies who share similar fitness goals and values. Lean on your support system for encouragement, motivation, and accountability during times of challenge or temptation.

10. Flexibility and Adaptability: Be flexible and adaptable in your approach to fitness and nutrition, and be willing to adjust your goals or strategies as needed to accommodate changes in your lifestyle, preferences, or circumstances.

By incorporating these tips into your daily routine, you can maintain your body sculpting results and enjoy a healthy, balanced lifestyle for years to come. Remember that consistency, patience, and self-care are key to long-term success.

Conclusion:

Congratulations on completing the SculptHer 12-week body sculpting plan! Remember, this journey is not just about physical transformation but also about embracing a healthier lifestyle and feeling confident in your own skin. Keep challenging yourself, stay consistent, and enjoy the incredible benefits of your hard work. You're unstoppable!

———-------

12 Week
"SculptHer"
Body Sculpt Plan for Women - Sample Program

Creating a 12-week body sculpting plan for women requires a combination of strength training, cardiovascular exercise, flexibility work, and proper nutrition. Remember to tailor the plan to individual fitness levels, goals, and any existing medical conditions.

Here's a generalized plan and sample program to build your own plan from:

Week 1-4: Foundation Building

Strength Training:
- Frequency: 2-3 times per week
- Focus: Full-body workouts targeting major muscle groups

Superset 1: Do Squats first, then Lunges, then rest 1 minute to 90 seconds between rounds.

- Squats: 3 sets of 10-12 reps
- Lunges: 3 sets of 10-12 reps per leg

Superset 2: Do Push-ups, then Bent-over Rows, then rest 1 minute to 90 seconds between rounds.
- Push-ups: 3 sets of 8-10 reps
- Bent-over rows: 3 sets of 10-12 reps

Superset 3: Do Planks, then Leg Raises, then rest 1 minute to 90 seconds between rounds.
- Planks: 3 sets, hold for 30-60 seconds
- Leg Raises: 3 sets of 10-12 reps

- Start with lighter weights and gradually increase as you get comfortable with the exercises.
- Add reps on the bodyweight exercises, or light weights such as ankle weights for leg raises, or weighted vests for push-ups and lunges.

Cardiovascular Exercise:
- Frequency: 3-5 times per week
- Duration: 20-30 minutes per session
- Choose activities you enjoy like brisk walking, jogging, cycling, or swimming.
- Incorporate different paces (easy, moderate, quick) for various times for an interval training effect. Example: walk for 2 minutes, jog for 1 minute, repeat 7 to 10 times.

Flexibility:
- Incorporate stretching exercises after workouts to improve flexibility and prevent injury.
- Focus on stretching major muscle groups like hamstrings, quadriceps, calves, chest, back, and shoulders.

Nutrition:
- Focus on balanced meals with lean proteins, complex carbohydrates, healthy fats, and plenty of fruits and vegetables.
- Stay hydrated by drinking plenty of water throughout the day.
- Aim for smaller, frequent meals to maintain energy levels and keep metabolism active.

Week 5-8: Intensification

Strength Training:
- Increase intensity by adding more weight or resistance.
- Incorporate workout circuits to increase calorie burn and muscle endurance.
- Example: Perform 3-6 exercises in a circuit, taking short breaks after rounds
- Alternate between upper, lower and core exercises within the circuit to allow brief rests for those areas within the circuit.

Squats: 4 sets of 10-12 reps

DB Chest Press: 4 sets of 10-12 reps
DB Lunges: 4 sets of 10-12 reps
Pulldowns or Cable Rows: 4 sets of 10-12 reps
Stability Ball or Floor Crunches: 4 sets of 10-12 reps
Russian Twists or Bicycle Crunches: 4 sets of 10-12 reps per side

Cardiovascular Exercise:
- Introduce more interval training to boost calorie burn and improve cardiovascular fitness.
- Alternate between high-intensity bursts and lower-intensity recovery periods during cardio sessions.
- Example: Sprints with Walking recovery periods, Sprinting 30 seconds with 2:30 to 3:30 of walking, repeating for 20-30 minutes based on your ability. This interval style can be applied to cycling/spinning, elliptical, rowing, and other cardio methods. Go between sprint efforts and easy pace efforts for the recovery times.

Flexibility:
- Continue with regular stretching sessions, focusing on deeper stretches to improve flexibility further.
- Consider incorporating activities like yoga or Pilates to enhance flexibility and core strength.

Nutrition:
- Monitor portion sizes and ensure a balance of nutrients to support energy levels and muscle recovery.
- Consider consulting with a nutritionist for personalized dietary guidance.

Week 9-12: Peak Performance

Strength Training:
- Incorporate more advanced exercises or variations to challenge muscles further.
- Focus on progressive overload by gradually increasing weights or resistance.
This will be a time to focus on Maximum Strength, a small change for a few weeks to lift heavier weights for less reps. Take more rest between sets as heavier weights need more recovery time. Maximum Strength workouts can be 2 days a week, with a Core day in between to help as a lighter recovery style workout. (Example: Monday/Friday as Strength days, Wednesday as a Core day)

Maximum Strength focus: 2 days per week
Squats or Deadlifts: 4 sets of 5-6 reps
Bench Press: 4 sets of 5-6 reps
DB 1 Arm Cleans: 4 sets of 5-6 reps per side
DB 1 Arm Rows: 4 sets of 5-6 reps per side

Core Focus: done between the two heavier strength sessions

Stability Ball Crunches: 3 sets of 12-15 reps
Leg Raises: 3 sets of 12-15 reps
Med Ball or DB Twists: 3 sets of 10-12 reps per side
Single Leg Deadlifts with DB or KB: 3 sets of 8-10 per side
Glute Bridges on Stability Ball: 3 sets of 10-12 reps
Standing Windmills: 3 sets of 4-5 reps per side

Cardiovascular Exercise:
- Mix up cardio routines to prevent plateaus and keep workouts challenging and enjoyable.
- Experiment with different activities or classes to keep motivation high.

Flexibility:
- Maintain consistency with stretching routines and explore advanced stretching techniques.
- Consider foam rolling or massage therapy to alleviate muscle tightness and improve recovery.

Nutrition:
- Fine-tune dietary habits based on progress and goals.
- Focus on nutrient-dense foods to support performance and recovery during the final weeks of
the program.

Additional Tips:
- Listen to your body and adjust workouts or rest days as needed to prevent overtraining and
injury.
- Track progress regularly, including measurements, strength gains, and overall fitness
improvements.
- Get adequate rest and prioritize sleep to support recovery and muscle growth.
- Stay motivated by setting realistic goals and celebrating achievements along the way.

Remember, consistency and dedication are key to achieving desired results. Always consult
with a healthcare professional before starting any new exercise or nutrition program, especially
if you have any underlying health conditions or concerns.

Discover more fitness strategies at https://rixfit5000.com and learn about the unique concept of
adding a simple workout finisher, and how a 30 day challenge along with it can add an extra
workout each week without finding more time for one!